Empowered Health

*Affirmations and reflections for
your health and wellness journey*

Constance C. Foreman, MD

ISBN: 979-8-9923540-0-3
First Edition

Published by
Beyond Clinic Walls Wellness, PLLC
info@beyondclinicwallswellness.com
www.beyondclinicwallswellness.com

Introduction

In 2021, I decided to embark on an entrepreneurial journey and started my first business: Beyond Clinic Walls Wellness, PLLC. Beyond Clinic Walls Wellness is a health education business that offers programming and speaking designed to provide the general public with accurate health information to make healthy living approachable and practical.

Sharing that tidbit might seem like an odd start to an affirmation book, but stay with me. I'm sure you remember that in 2021 we were still in the midst of a worldwide pandemic. And like many other people, I was forced to take a close look at my life. As a family medicine physician, I had been seeing patients virtually, while also caring for my mother who was diagnosed with SARS-CoV-2 (COVID-19) within the first weeks of the announcement of the pandemic. After nursing her back to health, I volunteered as a Navy Medical

Officer to go to Guam with the Navy Reserve and provided medical care to the USS Theodore Roosevelt after an outbreak of COVID-19 happened on the ship.

More than ever, my calling to help keep people healthy was loud and clear, but I knew that how I did this was evolving, both out of necessity and self-preservation. The stress and uncertainty of what we were all experiencing due to COVID-19 highlighted some of the shortcomings of our healthcare system and sparked something in me. The "post-pandemic world" was scary and I was faced with the reality of my own mortality. This realization inspired me to think hard about what I wanted in life, and I asked myself, "What can I do today to make my future a little brighter?"

The answer I came up with was to be intentional about carving out my own space in the world that reflected my beliefs and values. Beyond Clinic Walls Wellness is just that!

I want the world to know that being healthy is more than feeling good, numbers on a scale or even results from lab testing! In fact, even though I know it is important for people to have a primary care provider (my livelihood depends on it), the truth is that the majority of what is necessary for a person to stay healthy happens outside of the doctor's office. Beyond Clinic Walls Wellness is a business that helps me share my core values as a physician with the public on a smaller scale and now Empowered Health is something tangible that can go to infinity and beyond, planting seeds of positivity that will sprout and bloom into healthier, more confident individuals.

In this book, you'll find a collection of affirmations – some accompanied by short reflections – that will inspire and motivate you on your path to maintaining a healthy lifestyle. Each affirmation is designed to help you cultivate a mindset of resilience, determination, and self-love as you navigate the ups and downs of your health journey. Remember, you have the power to make your future a little brighter by creating the life and the health you desire.

I invite you to randomly flip through this book, read, and reflect. Let's continue the journey of healthy living!

Sincerely,

Dr. Constance

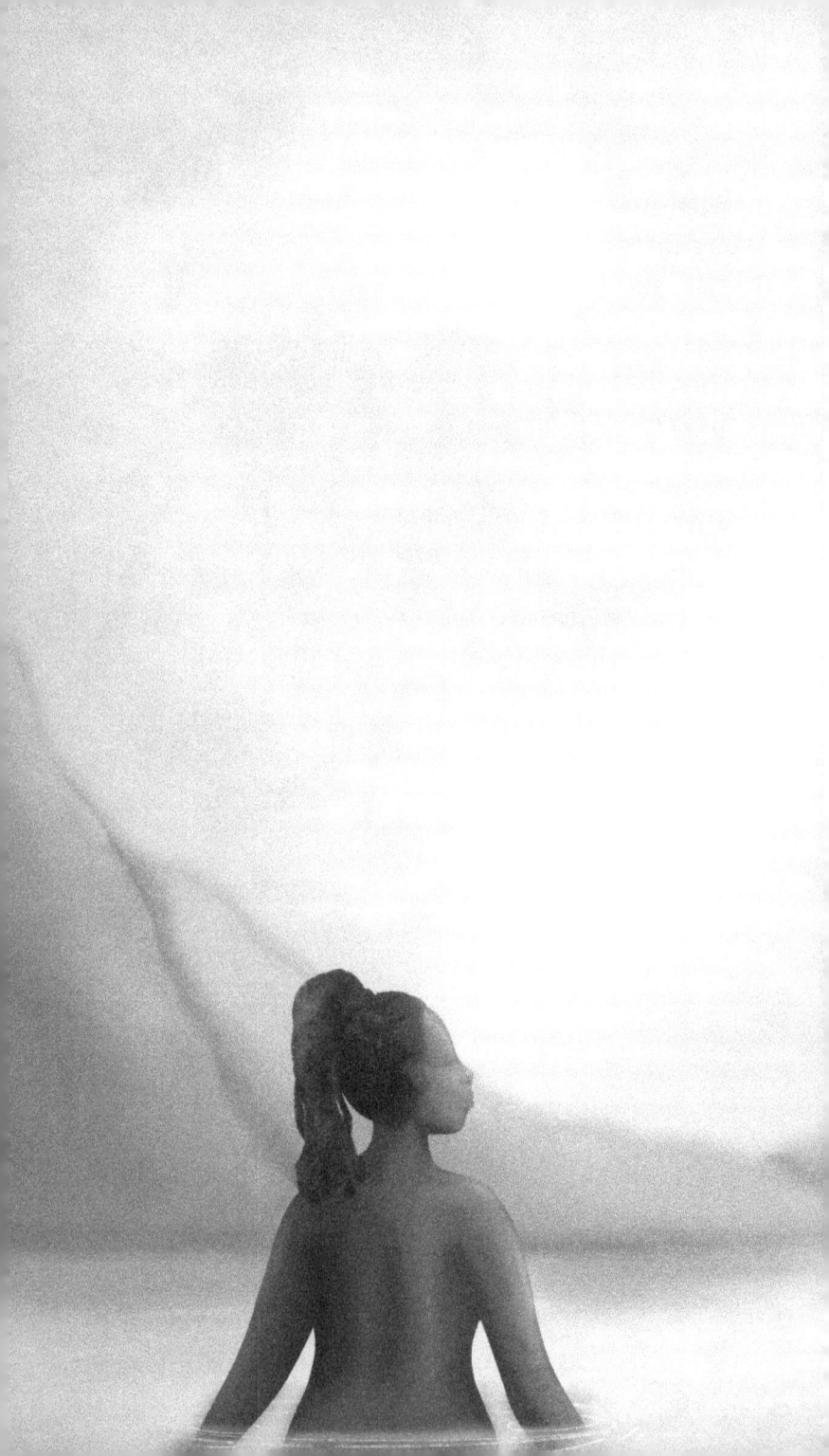

My being transcends my
health challenges.

I chose to live
the best life I can.

My health is more than numbers on a scale.

I will move my body because it feels good.

Being healthy is not a
chore for me but,
instead, a choice.

I have control
over my health.

I will commit to myself
by caring for my body.

My health is
my responsibility.

I am not my diagnosis.

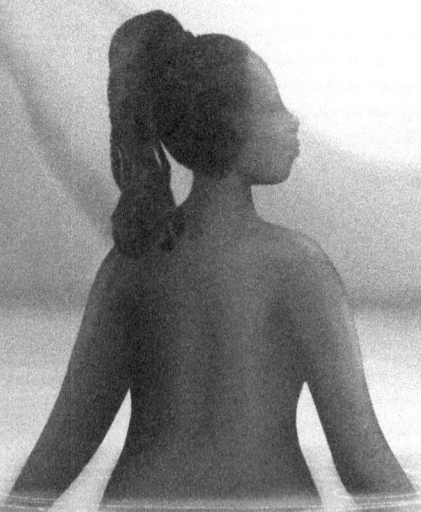

When we receive a new diagnosis, it is easy to become consumed by the implications that the diagnosis might have. In fact, we sometimes take a diagnosis, which is used to describe a disease, condition or injury, and use it to describe ourselves. When we do this, we connect our identity - who we are and how we see ourselves - with the condition itself. A condition that we are diagnosed with may affect how we live our lives, but it is not the totality of our being. I encourage you not to center your identity around any medical diagnosis you have; experience it, learn from it, but don't become it.

You are not your diagnosis.

My success is not based on a special diet.

When it comes to my health, I am the MVP!

There is power
in my words,
so I speak positively
about myself
and my health.

Food is not my enemy.

There is a purpose for
my life.

I can eat
my favorite foods
and still be healthy.

Sharing my goals with others not only empowers me but inspires others.

I will not be my own worst enemy.

My body is like a brick house and nothing can knock me down.

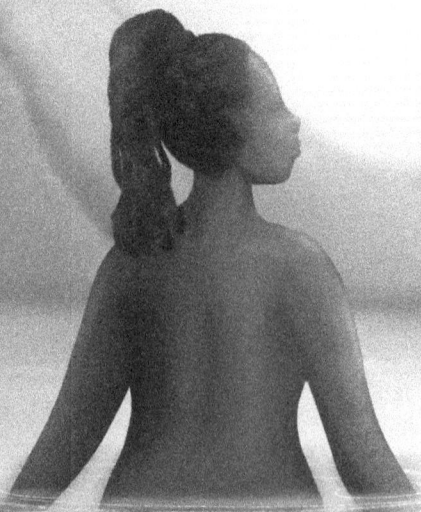

This affirmation evokes both beauty and strength. The Commodores hit song "Brick House" describes a smart, confident, and physically attractive woman. When I hear the term "brick house," it makes me want to strut around proudly and "let it all hang out," as the lyrics declare! In the fairy tale story of The Three Little Pigs, each of the three built their homes from different materials to protect themselves from the Big Bad Wolf. But only the brick house was successful because it was so strong. You are a brick house!

Not only is your body beautiful, but it is strong!

I value my emotional
well-being and
will not allow others
to weaponize
my self-worth.

It is OK for me to enjoy
my food.

I evaluate the relationships in my life and prioritize those that enhance my health.

I use the power of my mind to improve my health.

I am special, so I treat myself with care.

I will show up for myself today and everyday.

I am deserving of a
healthy body.

My body is
uniquely mine.

*I am open to
trying new things
to improve my health.*

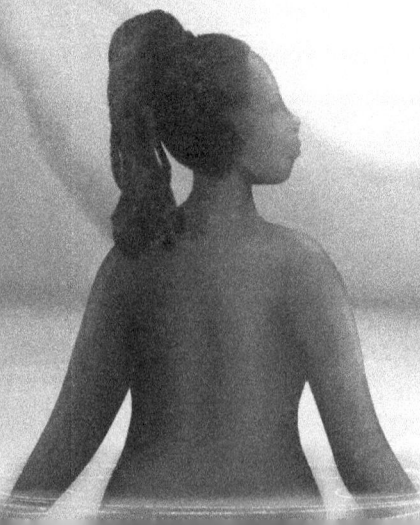

Many of us have heard the phrase "insanity is doing the same thing and expecting a different result." Consistency and commitment are important, but literally doing the same things everyday when it is not resulting in a desired outcome is counterproductive. This means that you might have to try some new things to see positive improvements in your health. This can mean a different way of cooking, eliminating behaviors that don't serve you, and even changing environments.

Be open to the possibilities of the new and unfamiliar.

I resist the urge
to compare my body
to others.

All aspects of my health
are important –
mental, physical,
emotional and spiritual.

I celebrate all of my wins, big and small.

I am worthy of love.

I focus on what feels good to my body.

I love and appreciate my body.

I will make good
decisions about
my health.

I will be intentional about
physical exercise.

*I can live a fulfilling life
in spite of my limitations*

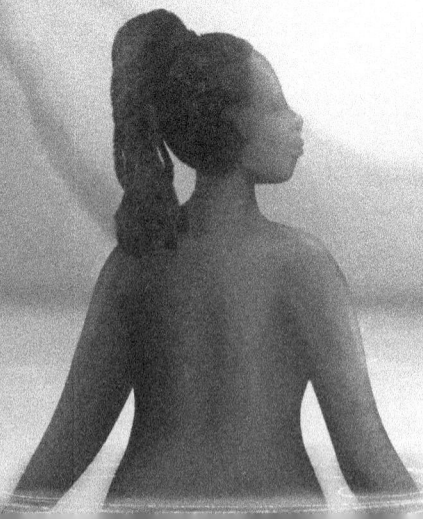

Why is it that we like to create so many boxes for ourselves? In a world in which freedom is one of the most sought-after states of being, we still find ways to restrict ourselves. There are certainly situations in which avoiding substances, food, and particular activities might be vital, but there are so many other choices that we can make in spite of special circumstances. There are some things that we cannot change about our lives but there are a few we can and we owe it to ourselves to spend a little time cultivating the behaviors and interventions that allow us to live a fulfilling life emotionally and physically.

We might have limits but our potential is limitless!

I trust my body to tell
me what it needs.

I will not sabotage my
efforts.

I am the curator of
positive outcomes
in my life.

I build healthy
relationships with
people around me.

My body is perfect
as it is.

Investing in my health is
a profitable investment.

I strive for progress and not perfection.

My body, mind, and spirit are in harmony.

Even when I feel that I have
fallen off the train
of healthy living,
it is OK because the next
train won't leave the station
without me.

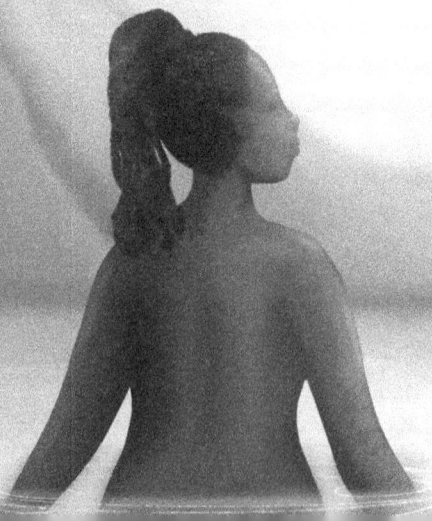

You might be familiar with the phrase 'when you fall off the horse you get back on' but I think a train is a more fitting analogy for resilience especially for our health and wellness journey. Trains can cross long distances and usually make multiple stops. Trains also have schedules that get repeated over a predetermined period. Our health journey will span the duration of our lives and may even stop us in our tracks (pun intended) at times. Even though we might have to take time to find our way and restructure our habits, we have the opportunity to step off the metaphorical platform at the station and back onto the train car, ready for the next station towards a better life.

We determine the distance we go, the stops we make, and the schedule we keep for a healthy life.

My good health comes
from practicing
good habits.

Nurturing myself
is not selfish.

I treat my body like
the temple that is it.

My mind holds
deep wisdom.

My healthy self is an asset to this world.

Good food, good sleep, and good exercise are necessities and not luxuries.

Loving myself allows me to love others more fully.

I am thriving, mentally and physically.

*I am ready for
a healthy life.*

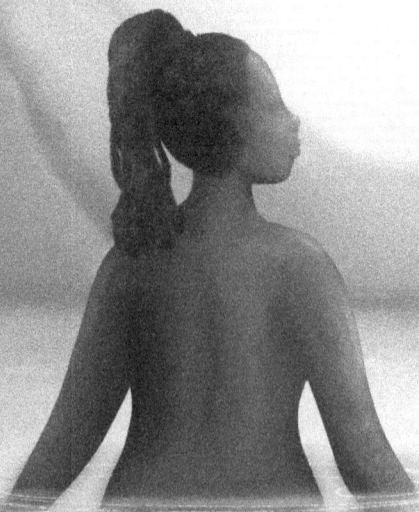

Half of the battle to achieve any goal is intentionality and readiness to change. The Stages of Change module is a tool used to determine a person's motivation to make a particular behavior change. As a physician, I use The Stages of Change module to assess my patients' motivation for behavioral changes that would benefit their health. The first step is called Precontemplation. At this stage, a person has not yet acknowledged the problem or has no interest in changing it. I know that you are past the Precontemplation stage because you purchased this book. You have thought about your health and have recognized that some of the things that you were doing before do not serve you. Once you have acknowledged a problem or concern over time, you start to prepare to make the change until one day you are ready to spring into action.

I believe that you are ready! Do you?

Healing is possible
for me.

My body is strong
and capable.

I have abundant energy.

It is easy for me
to eat well.

Food is a tool
to nourish my body.

I feel best when I am
active.

I am proud of myself for caring for my body.

I rest when I need it.

*I work seamlessly
with health professionals
to improve my health.*

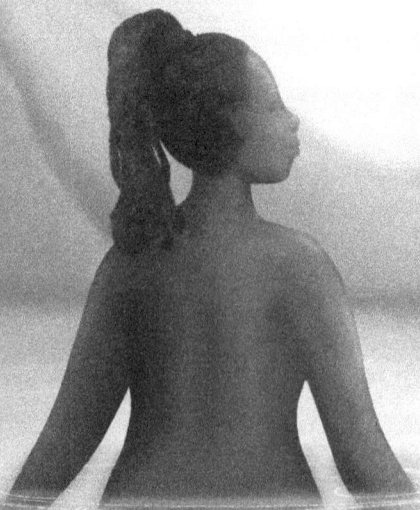

When you enter the examination room of any physician or other healthcare professional, you should feel like you are walking into an important strategy meeting for a big project with a trusted business partner. You and the provider should communicate well and be on the same page about your health goals so that you can effectively "seal the deal."

Strive for meaningful conversations that lead to impactful changes in your health where you are able to give information to the provider and receive feedback.

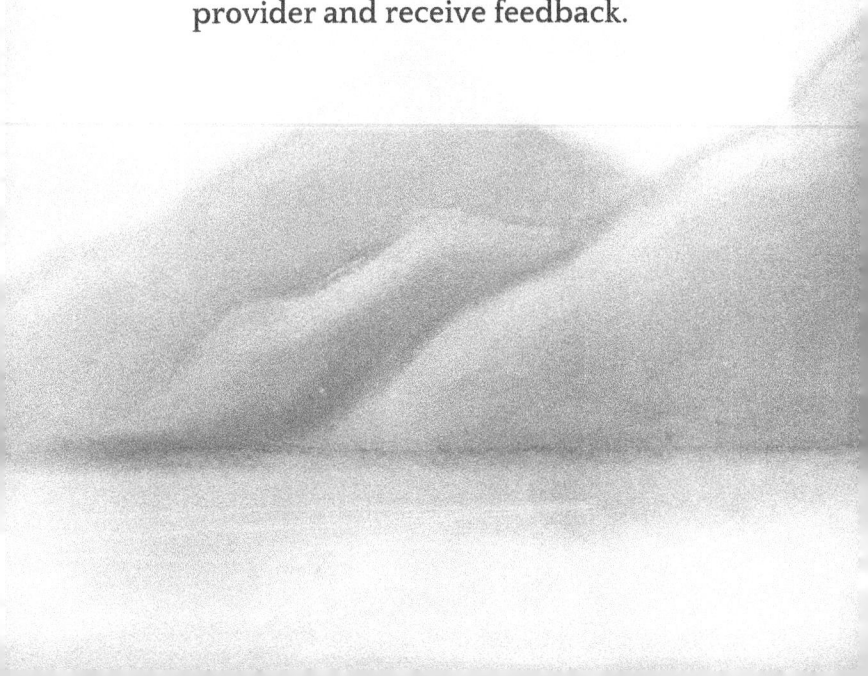

My mind is at peace.

I am only in competition
with the person I was
yesterday.

I love myself enough to live a healthy lifestyle.

I exercise to be fit, not skinny.

I am more worthy
than I realize.

I have my health,
therefore I have hope.

My healthy outer
appearance starts
from within.

I cannot control
everything, but
I can control my choices.

*I can eat well
without eating perfectly.*

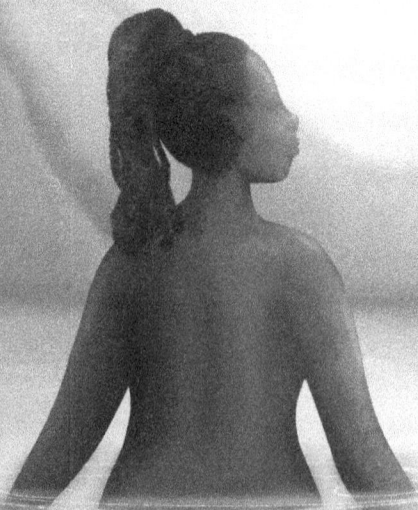

What is the "perfect" way of eating? Is it Keto, Paleo, intermittent fasting, the Mediterranean diet, vegan or some other dietary recommendation? Well, the truth is that there is no such thing as perfect. As we prepare our meals and snacks, we should focus on eating well, which means a balanced approach to eating. Some days we may have junk food or alcohol, but it's OK because these items can be a part of a balanced and fulfilling diet. When you combine vegetables, fruits, whole grains, and other nutritious foods with your Oreos, Cheetos and margaritas you have cracked the code!

Strive to eat well, not perfectly.

I am falling in love
with caring for my body.

I am healing myself by
making better choices.

I am doing enough.

I am confident that I can achieve my goals.

My feelings matter.

I am resilient.

I am getting stronger
everyday.

Making nourishing
decisions is easy for me.

*Being healthy is
not simply the
absence of sickness.*

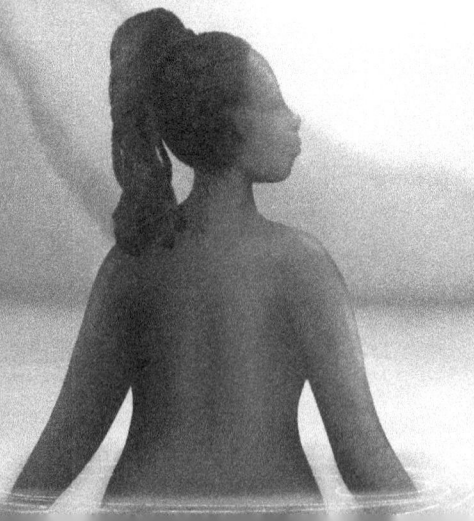

How we define "health" affects how we manage it. If you think that being healthy means never experiencing a health challenge, then you are doomed from the start. You are only human and your body is susceptible to illness and injury; but, you are also a miraculous creature with the ability to heal and improve! I like to think of being healthy as being able to prevent and/or overcome a health challenge. While you might have received a diagnosis, it does not define you (remember there was an affirmation for this)! With the help of appropriate interventions, we are able to restore our mental and physical health which allows us to effectively care for ourselves and experience joy.

Illness or disease may create a new normal for you but it is possible to find your way back to balance.

I focus on the present.

My body likes trying
new exercises.

I am not my fears.

Exercise makes me a
happier person.

I strive to find balance in how I live my life.

I am building the foundation for wellness.

I try my best every day.

I cannot go back and change the beginning, but I do have control of the ending.

I am not alone on my health journey.

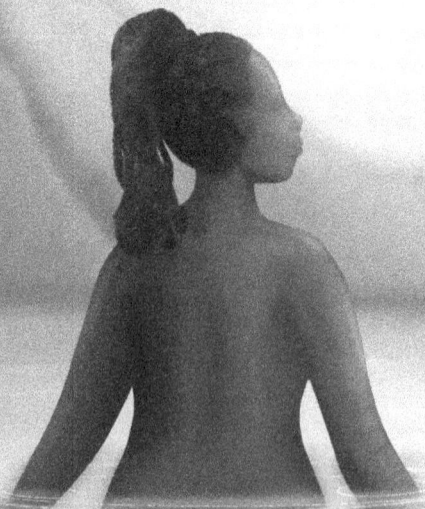

It is not uncommon to feel alone when we are experiencing health challenges. It can be difficult to connect with people or find a sense of belonging because what is happening to our body feels so foreign. The truth is that you are not alone! There are billions of people in the world and there is at least one who is going through something similar to you. More importantly, there is someone out there who can support you through your journey.

**As you continue on your journey,
know that you are not alone and that
there is power in building community.**

I speak to my body
with positive intent.

My environment supports
my health goals.

Water gives life
to my body.

I will not overindulge in
things that can harm me.

I focus on
my healed self.

My imagination helps
create my reality.

I say yes to things that support holistic wellness.

I consume positive information and interactions.

I learn from the health challenges of my family but do not make them my own.

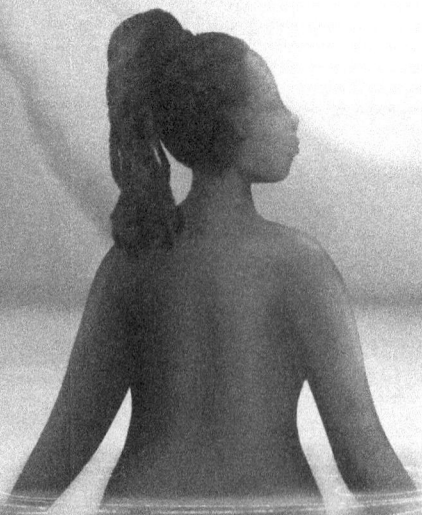

Our genetic makeup is something that we cannot hide from. It is important to be aware of it and use that knowledge to prevent health complications as best we can. However, as we embrace the truth of our family history we have to avoid the urge to yield to them and focus more on our own health. In fact, some of the health challenges experienced by our family members are actually a reflection of their behaviors and not genetics. This strengthens the need to exhibit positive behaviors and live as a change agent for your family tree.

Root your family tree in positivity and help shape its growth.

I choose myself.

When I stay in my lane,
there is never traffic.

The world needs
people like me.

I protect my body
by making
healthy decisions.

My body is amazing.

I find ways to
manage my stress to
positively impact
my health.

I give my attention
to things that
improve my health.

When I daydream,
I see my healthiest self.

*Sickness is a trigger
to help me
back to wellness.*

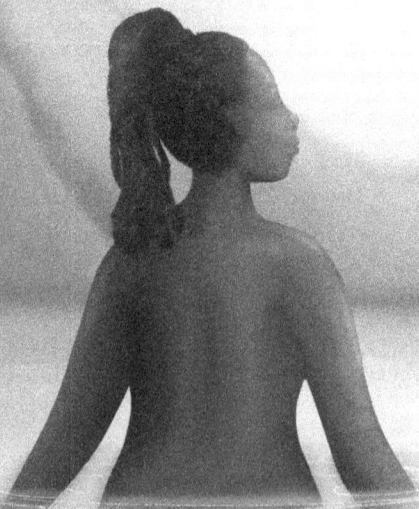

Previously, I encouraged us all to affirm the fact that being healthy is not simply the absence of sickness. This affirmation reinforces that fact. When something happens to us that negatively impacts our health it is an opportunity to make a change that is going to lead to a better outcome.

Don't let your illness prevent you from pursuing wellness but, instead, inspire it.

I say no to things
that don't serve
my wellness journey.

Sunshine feeds my soul
and
strengthens my body.

I understand that
sharing my emotions is
not a sign of weakness.

I talk the talk
and walk the walk.

Today,
I choose to be positive.

The evolution of my
self-care is fulfillment.

I am the leader
of my healthcare team.

Fun is a priority
in my healthy life.

*I am honest with myself
about my health.*

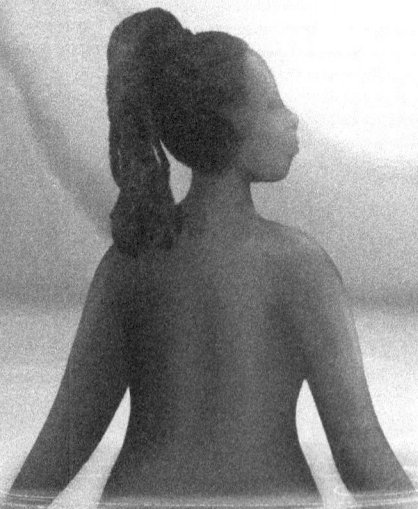

Honesty is the best policy, right? Usually, we are sharing this sentiment related to our interactions with others but what about having the same energy and being self-aware about how we treat ourselves?

Take the time to appraise your health and your efforts at improving it, because if you lie to yourself, you're lying to the most important person in your life.

I support my wellness
with positive uplifting
perspectives.

I exercise
to honor my body.

I am a magnet for
healthy and uplifting
energy.

I will find strength
in my challenges.

I don't have to be extreme about my health, just consistent.

I am creating a body that I enjoy living in.

I will find healthcare
professionals that
genuinely care about me.

I advocate for
my health needs
in a productive way.

I will eat, drink, and be merry without fear of my health.

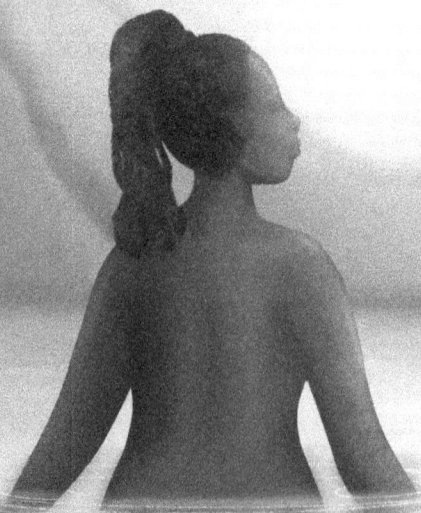

Living without fear does not mean that there are no consequences to what we do. Choosing to eat and drink without fear is a way to take ownership of your experiences, as well as acknowledge the need to be intentional about finding balance in the things you partake in. Find strength in the knowledge that you gain about your body and mind.

Put your fear on the shelf and instead use your concern to mold the decisions that you make everyday.

I am doing
the right things
for my health.

There is always hope
to do and be better.

I am making way for
unprecedented success
in my life.

My heart and mind
are open to
my healthiest self.

The perfect moment
to be healthy is now.

The rest of my life
is going to be incredible.

Who I am
helps me achieve
my wildest dreams.

My perspective
is important.

I am not scared
of my diagnosis.

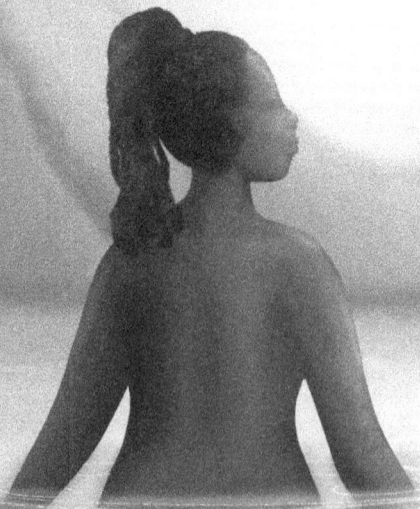

This is a loaded affirmation, but a very important one. If we are in the dark about something, then we are powerless against it. Fear often prevents us from exploring the shadows of our existence. If we allow fear to paralyze us, we are also limiting our progress toward wellness. By embracing our diagnoses, we can learn more about them and be better equipped to shape the experiences that we have.

Be brave!

I will do away
with decisions that
do not support self–care.

Being positive never hurt
anyone.

I am good at taking care
of myself.

I am better
than I used to be.

I choose to learn from
my negative experiences.

I am rooting
for myself and the
people around me.

I deserve everything
I desire.

I am unaffected by
the judgment of others.

My weight does not determine my joy.

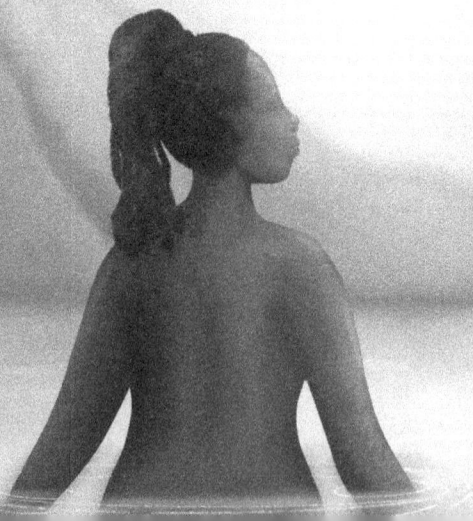

Since the late 19th century weight has been a popular topic in magazines, other media sources and, of course, at the doctors office. While weight has been linked to certain medical conditions, any focus we make at improving our health should be holistic and not overemphasize one piece of the healthy living puzzle.

No matter what the scale says when you step on it, you can live a fulfilling life!

I will be accountable
for my behaviors.

I am healing
more and more
every day.

I am in control of
my health, my health
does not control me.

I love the person I see
when I look
in the mirror.

My body can achieve
what my mind believes.

Becoming my healthiest
self will require patience.

My self-control starts
with self-awareness.

I embody love for myself
that makes
being healthy easy.

I do not have to be miserable to be healthy.

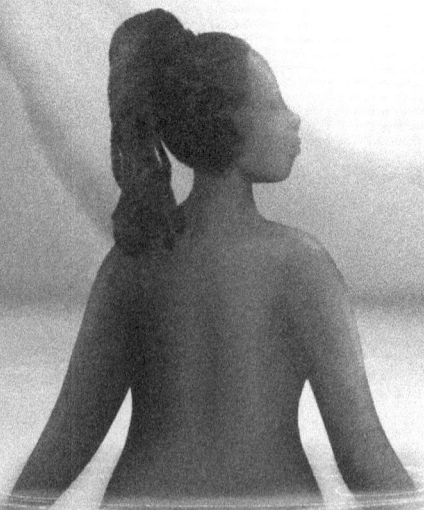

I have noticed a trend in the health and wellness industry that focuses on restriction and all the things we shouldn't do to be healthy. I'm a doctor and this approach is overwhelming to me, so I can only imagine how the average person might feel. When we think about our wellness, we should think less about what we have to give up and more about what we will gain with our new behaviors. Yes, you might have to change some things, but you DO NOT have to sacrifice easy living or enjoyable food!

Being healthy is about living so remember to do just that – LIVE!

I choose thoughts
of total wellness.

I am grateful
for my body.

I support my wellness
by minimizing negativity.

I will protect my health
at all costs.

It takes more than prescription medications and supplements to maintain my health.

I am gentle with myself as I improve my health.

I will focus on
aspects of my health
that I have control over.

I avoid behaviors that
increase my risk for
chronic medical
conditions.

I acknowledge that the internet is an amazing tool, but it cannot answer all of my health questions.

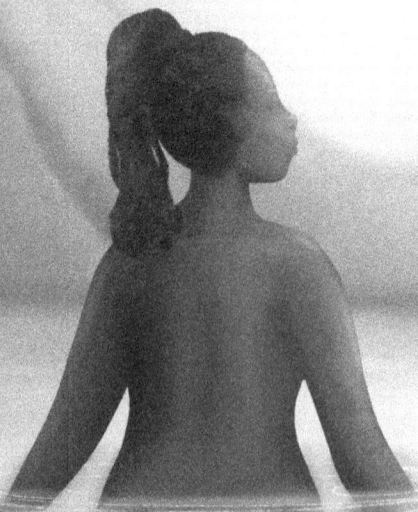

This affirmation is personal for me and I had to slide it in. As a millennial, I am completely on board with advanced technology and use parts of the internet for my medical practice and personal health concerns. It is a good way to orient myself and often a way to find starting points for conversations related to an array of topics. However, we have to find balance in how we use the internet and the insight that can be provided by healthcare professionals who know us.

Don't let things that you read on the internet trump the advice that you receive in the healthcare setting. Instead, use the information to enhance your healthcare experience.

I do not let the words and actions of others prevent me from being my best self.

I do not live in the past but, instead, focus on my future self.

I will seek out
understanding of my
health concerns
and not be afraid
to ask questions.

I practice
health behaviors that are
safe for my body.

I care about my health because I want to live a long and fulfilling life.

It does not matter what I do to exercise as long as I do it consistently.

I decide what a healthy body looks like for me.

I release all guilt and shame about my body.

Discussing health as a family will strengthen future generations.

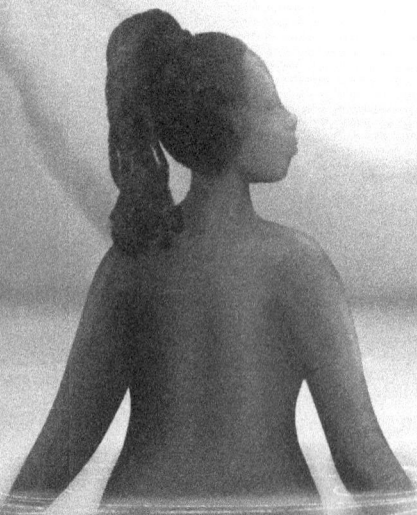

The beautiful thing about knowledge is that it is an asset that can be easily shared. While knowledge is valuable for ourselves, we can give it freely to whomever we'd like to - and why not share with our family? The individuals we share a blood connection to are sometimes susceptible to the conditions we possess and vice versa. By discussing these things freely, we are not only fostering a welcoming environment in which people feel safe to be vulnerable, but we are setting the groundwork for learning valuable information on how we can better care for each other, make life-changing decisions for better health and even prevent unwanted conditions for future generations.

Be bold, be supportive and have important health conversations with your family if, and while, you can.

I am happy to be alive.

I enjoy seeing
how healthy habits
improve my life.

I make time to care for
my mental health.

I have all of the energy
I need to accomplish
my goals.

I work at my own pace
and listen to
my body's needs.

I adapt my lifestyle
to fit my health needs.

I choose to act proactively towards a healthier life.

Strong is who I am.

I give my body permission to change.

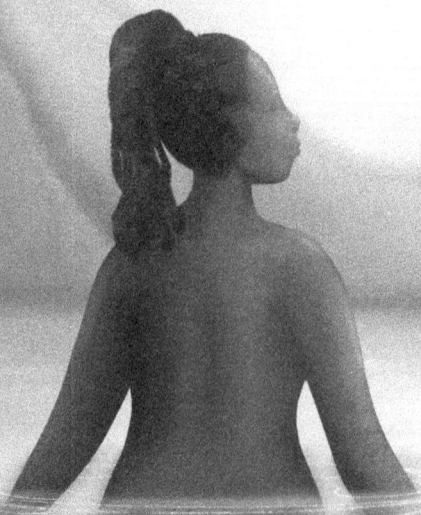

The Greek philosopher Heraclitus is credited with the idea that the only thing constant in life is change. With every year that passes in our lives we are growing mentally and emotionally and as this happens our bodies are slowly transforming as well. This is the natural order of life and there is beauty in the process.

Give yourself permission to morph and embrace who you are becoming.

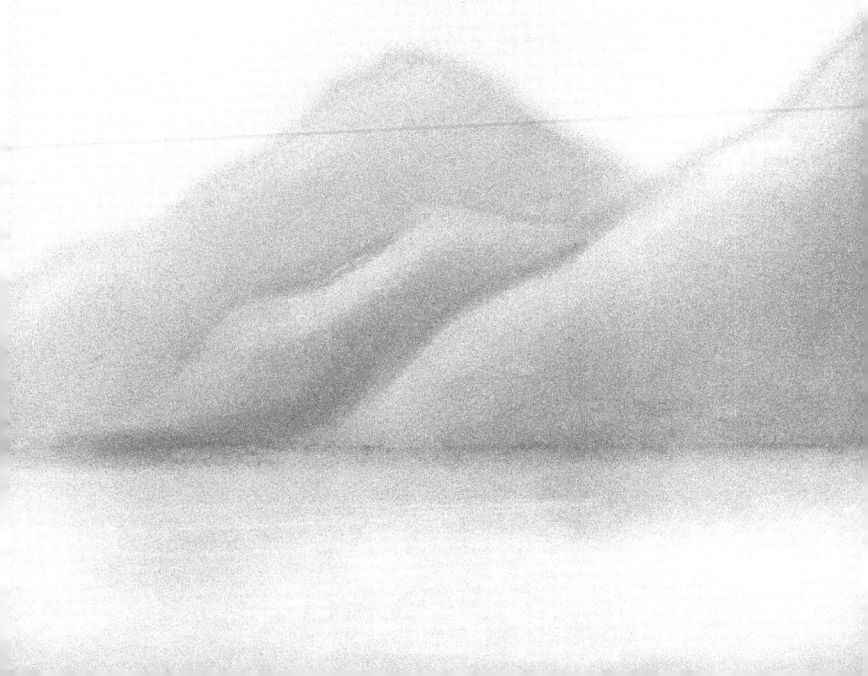

I accept my body
and acknowledge
the beauty it holds.

I have hope about
the future of my health.

I am taking small steps
towards success.

The choices I make
are consistent with
my future goals.

I like creating
healthy habits that
I will use for the
rest of my life.

I take time to rest
because it helps me
become mentally and
physically stronger

I am a beacon of vitality.

I am doing all that I can
to keep my health
under control.

I am wise enough to know when to seek help for my medical concerns.

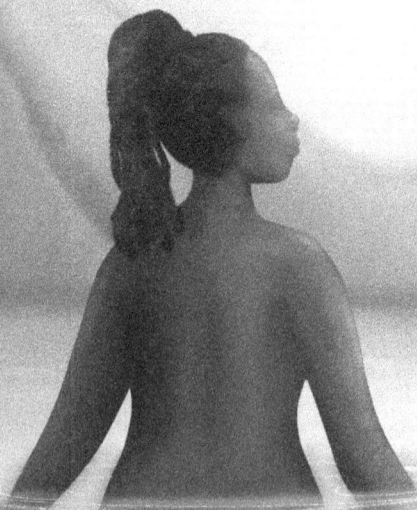

We all have that one stubborn friend or family member. Actually, you might be that stubborn friend or family member and that's OK! Stubborn people often get a bad reputation, but independence is the essence of who they are. They are determined to find their own way in their own time. It is admirable to be self sufficient, strong-willed, and self-reliant, but even the strongest people sometimes need help. Be tenacious, but not at the expense of your health.

You have the wisdom to submit to your needs and ask for help. Your health depends on it.

I am proud of the effort
I put towards
being healthy today.

I wake up every day
with good health at the
forefront of my mind.

I have a
deep appreciation
for myself.

My body is
my most precious asset.

The state of
my body reflects
the peace of my mind.

I will learn
to say yes to myself
even if that means
saying no to others.

I am bold
about asserting
my health needs.

Even in the
face of adversity,
I will keep
a positive outlook.

*I pay the cost
to be the boss.*

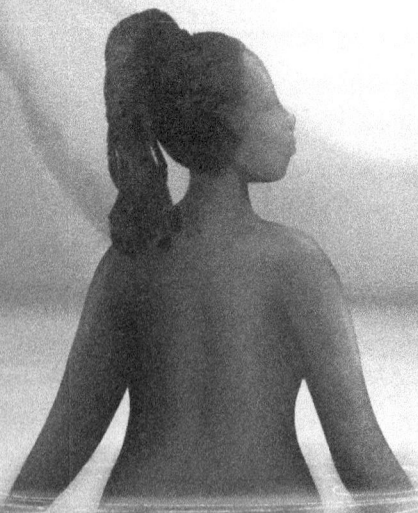

I cannot take the credit for this affirmation. This statement is brought to you by my mother and I have taken ownership of it. When I was a child and I objected to something my mom asked me to do, she would say "Excuse me, but I pay the cost to be the boss." Of course, I was always annoyed when she'd say this but it was burned into my memory and resurfaced when I started practicing medicine. You see, when my mom would say this she was reminding me of the authority she had in our household and the efforts that she made to take care of me. At that time, it was a way for her to disarm me but now I use it to empower patients and clients. You have the freedom to make the final decisions about your health!

Determine what is important to you and how you want to shape your future and own it. You're the boss!

Conclusion

Your health journey is a unique and deeply personal one, but you don't have to travel it alone. With the power of affirmations and reflections for inspiration shared in this book, you have the tools you need to cultivate a mindset of empowerment, resilience, and self-love.

Remember, true health is not just about the absence of disease but about thriving in every aspect of your life.

Embrace the journey, believe in yourself, and know that you are capable of achieving the vibrant health and happiness you deserve.

About the Author

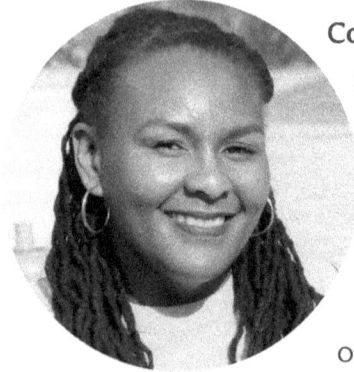

Constance Foreman, MD a Maryland native, discovered her passion for science and service early, blending a love for exploration with a drive to make a difference. After earning her Bachelor of Arts in Biology from St. Mary's College of Maryland, she served with AmeriCorps VISTA before pursuing advanced medical education, earning a Master of Medical Science from Hampton University and her Doctor of Medicine degree from Eastern Virginia Medical School. A Navy Reserve officer and Family Medicine physician in Wilmington, NC, Dr. Foreman is also the founder of Beyond Clinic Walls Wellness, a health education and speaking business dedicated to empowering individuals to achieve lasting wellness through practical lifestyle changes.

For inquiries on speaking engagements, health education content and other ways to work with Dr. Foreman contact:

www.beyondclinicwallswellness.com

info@beyondclinicwallswellness.com

(910) 679-6419

Or scan the QR Code to connect!

About the Illustrator

JaVon L. Townsend, LCSW-C is a narrative artist whose work centers love, joy, and connection. She is a storyteller who uses words and images to help celebrate the beauty and full humanity, primarily, of Black and Brown people. JaVon is formally trained as a Licensed Clinical Social Worker, supporting people in re-telling their own stories through utilizing the creative arts in healing work. She sees her artwork as an extension of this practice, seeking to connect the personal with the universal. JaVon was selected to be part of the inaugural cohort of the We Need Diverse Books Black Creatives Mentorship Program in 2023. She is the author and illustrator of "Peaceful Plants: A Mindfulness Coloring Book."

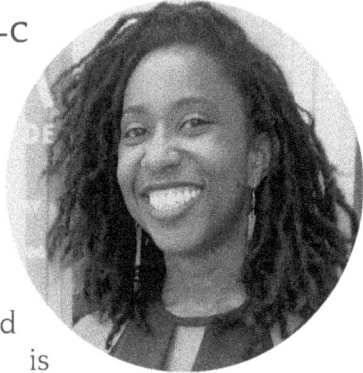

For inquiries on illustration, self-publishing consultation or editing, speaking engagements, or other ways to work with JaVon, contact:

javontownsendart@gmail.com

View more of JaVon's work @javonmakesart on Youtube and Instagram
Or scan the QR code to connect!